No Carb Food List

Elevate Your Cooking Game: Discovering the Endless Possibilities of No-Carb Foods

McDonnell B. Young

Table of Contents

Introduction

In a city filled with endless food options, Alex had always found himself grappling with a diet that seemed to spiral out of control. Despite numerous attempts at various eating plans, he struggled with persistent fatigue, weight gain, and constant cravings. The search for a solution seemed never-ending until he stumbled upon the "No Carb Food List" guide.

Alex was skeptical at first. Could a simple list really be the answer to his problems? His curiosity was piqued, so he decided to give it a try. What he discovered within those pages was nothing short of transformative.

The guide began with a clear and comprehensive explanation of the no-carb concept, demystifying what seemed like an overwhelming dietary restriction. It detailed how eliminating carbs could lead to increased energy, improved mental clarity, and weight loss. The guide didn't just preach; it provided a well-researched and easy-to-understand rationale behind the no-carb approach.

The heart of the guide was its meticulously curated food lists. The "Foods to Eat" section introduced Alex to a variety of delicious and satisfying options he had never considered before. From succulent cuts of beef and flavorful seafood to rich, creamy cheeses and nutrient-dense leafy greens, the guide made it clear that a no-carb diet was not about deprivation but about enjoying high-quality, flavorful foods. Each category was thoughtfully organized, making meal planning a breeze.

Alex was equally impressed with the "Foods to Avoid" section. It was clear and precise, listing not only what to stay away from but also why those foods could hinder his progress. This section empowered Alex to make informed choices, avoiding the pitfalls that had previously derailed his attempts at healthier eating.

One of the guide's standout features was its practical advice on adhering to a no-carb diet. With helpful tips on meal planning, snacking wisely, and dining out, Alex felt supported and equipped to make lasting changes. The sample meal plans provided inspiration and variety, ensuring he never felt bored or deprived.

The guide also addressed common challenges and answered frequently asked questions, providing reassurance and practical solutions. It was evident that the guide was crafted with empathy and a deep understanding of the struggles faced by those new to a no-carb lifestyle.

In the end, Alex's transformation was profound. With the "No Carb Food List" guide in hand, he experienced a renewed sense of vitality and well-being. The guide wasn't just a list; it was a gateway to a healthier, more fulfilling life.

For anyone struggling with the complexities of diet and nutrition, the "No Carb Food List" guide offers a clear, practical, and empowering solution. It's not just a purchase; it's an investment in a brighter, healthier future.

Understanding the No Carb Concept

The no-carb concept revolves around eliminating carbohydrates from one's diet to achieve specific health goals, such as weight loss, improved energy levels, or better metabolic control. Carbohydrates, found in a wide array of foods including grains, fruits, and vegetables, are typically the body's primary source of energy. However, the idea behind a no-carb diet is to shift the body's energy reliance from carbohydrates to fats and proteins, which can lead to various health benefits.

Understanding the role of carbohydrates in the body is crucial to grasp the no-carb concept fully. Carbs are broken down into glucose, which is used for immediate energy or stored as glycogen in the liver and muscles. By reducing or eliminating carb intake, the body begins to use stored fat as its primary energy source through a process known as ketosis. This metabolic state can result in significant weight loss and improved fat-burning efficiency.

The no-carb approach is not just about cutting out obvious sources of carbs like bread, pasta, and sugary snacks. It also involves being vigilant about hidden carbs in processed foods and condiments, which can undermine the effectiveness of the diet. Consequently, adhering strictly to a no-carb diet requires a keen eye on food labels and ingredient lists to avoid inadvertently consuming carbohydrates.

Adopting a no-carb diet can also have implications for overall health and well-being. Many proponents of the diet report experiencing enhanced mental clarity and sustained energy levels, as the body becomes more adept at using fat for fuel. This shift can help stabilize blood sugar levels, reducing the risk of insulin resistance and type 2 diabetes.

One of the challenges of a no-carb diet is ensuring that nutritional needs are still met. With the exclusion of carbs, it's vital to focus on consuming sufficient proteins and healthy fats to maintain muscle mass and overall health. Foods such as lean meats, fish, eggs, and high-fat dairy products become primary staples in a no-carb regimen, providing essential nutrients without the carb content.

While the no-carb diet can be highly effective for many, it's important to approach it with a balanced perspective. It's crucial to listen to one's body and make adjustments as needed to ensure that the diet remains sustainable and healthful. Consulting with a healthcare professional or a registered dietitian can help tailor the diet to individual needs and address any potential nutritional gaps.

In summary, the no-carb concept involves a significant dietary shift that eliminates carbohydrates to promote fat burning and improve overall health. It requires careful planning and a thorough understanding of food sources to ensure adherence and effectiveness. By focusing on protein and fat-rich foods while avoiding hidden carbs, individuals can harness the benefits of a no-carb diet, achieving their health goals and potentially experiencing a renewed sense of vitality.

Benefits of a No Carb Diet

A no-carb diet offers numerous benefits that extend beyond simple weight loss. By significantly reducing or eliminating carbohydrates from your diet, you can experience a substantial boost in energy levels. Without the constant fluctuations in blood sugar levels that come from consuming carbs, your energy remains stable throughout the day, reducing feelings of fatigue and lethargy. This steady energy can enhance your productivity and overall mood, leading to a more balanced and invigorating lifestyle.

The no-carb approach can also lead to improved mental clarity and cognitive function. Carbohydrates, particularly those from high-glycemic foods, can cause brain fog and decreased concentration. By removing these carbs, the brain relies more on ketones produced from fats, which can offer a more consistent and clearer cognitive performance. This mental sharpness can be particularly beneficial in high-demand situations, such as work or academic pursuits.

Another significant advantage of a no-carb diet is its impact on weight management. Without the intake of carbohydrates, your body begins to burn stored fat for energy, leading to more efficient fat loss. This metabolic shift, known as ketosis, helps reduce body fat percentage and supports lean muscle mass. As a result, many individuals find it easier to maintain a healthy weight or achieve their desired weight loss goals.

In addition to aiding weight loss, a no-carb diet can also contribute to better heart health. By cutting out high-carb, processed foods and sugars, you reduce the risk of developing cardiovascular issues. This dietary change helps lower triglyceride levels and improve cholesterol profiles, which are critical for reducing the risk of heart disease. With a focus on healthy fats and lean proteins, the diet supports overall cardiovascular well-being.

Digestive health is another area that benefits from a no-carb diet. Carbohydrates, especially from refined grains and sugary foods, can contribute to digestive discomfort and irregularity. By eliminating these sources of carbs, you may experience improved digestion and reduced symptoms like bloating and gas. The guide's emphasis on whole, nutrient-dense foods ensures that you're getting essential vitamins and minerals without the digestive drawbacks of processed carbs.

Moreover, a no-carb diet can help stabilize mood and manage cravings. The elimination of sugar and refined carbs reduces the likelihood of mood swings and irritability, which are often linked to blood sugar spikes and crashes. By focusing on proteins and healthy fats, the diet helps keep hunger and cravings in check, leading to more consistent mood and satisfaction with meals.

Ultimately, the benefits of a no-carb diet are substantial and multifaceted, affecting energy levels, mental clarity, weight management, heart health, digestive comfort, and overall mood. The "No Carb Food List" guide is an essential tool in achieving these benefits, providing a clear and practical approach to dietary choices that support a healthier, more balanced lifestyle.

How to Use This Book

When embarking on a no-carb diet, the "No Carb Food List" book serves as a valuable tool to guide you through every step of the process. Start by familiarizing yourself with the core principles outlined in the early sections. These foundational concepts explain the rationale behind eliminating carbohydrates from your diet and highlight the benefits you can expect, such as improved energy levels and better overall health. Understanding these principles is crucial for making informed decisions and maintaining motivation throughout your dietary journey.

As you delve into the book, pay close attention to the comprehensive lists of foods to eat and foods to avoid. The detailed sections on foods you can enjoy include a diverse range of options, from various types of meat and seafood to specific cheeses and oils. These lists are designed to help you create balanced and satisfying meals without the confusion of sorting through countless labels. By focusing on these recommended foods, you'll be able to build a diet that is both nutritious and enjoyable.

The guide's section on foods to avoid is equally important. This part of the book outlines what to steer clear of, providing clear explanations as to why certain items, such as bread, pasta, and sugary snacks, should be eliminated from your diet. Understanding the reasons behind these restrictions helps you make better choices and avoid common pitfalls that could impede your progress. This knowledge empowers you to navigate grocery stores and restaurants with confidence.

To make the transition to a no-carb diet smoother, the book offers practical advice on meal planning and preparation. It includes strategies for organizing your weekly meals, ensuring that you have a variety of no-carb options available. This guidance is particularly useful for preventing the monotony of eating the same foods repeatedly and for avoiding the temptation of high-carb alternatives. Embrace the sample meal plans provided to inspire your cooking and make the dietary shift more manageable.

In addition to meal planning, the guide addresses how to handle social situations and dining out. It provides tips on how to stick to your no-carb diet while eating at restaurants or attending social gatherings. This practical advice ensures that you can maintain your dietary goals without feeling restricted or isolated. By following these strategies, you can enjoy social interactions without compromising your commitment to a no-carb lifestyle.

The troubleshooting and FAQs section of the book is an invaluable resource for addressing any challenges or questions that arise as you adapt to your new diet. Whether you encounter issues with cravings, meal variety, or understanding certain dietary principles, this section offers solutions and clarifications to help you stay on track. The support provided here can make the difference between a temporary diet change and a long-lasting lifestyle adjustment.

Lastly, as you continue using the book, take advantage of the glossary of terms and additional resources included at the end. These tools can help clarify any unfamiliar concepts and provide further reading for a deeper understanding of the no-carb approach. By integrating this knowledge into your daily routine, you'll enhance your ability to maintain a successful no-carb diet and achieve the health benefits you're aiming for.

Chapter 1: No Carb Food Essentials

What Constitutes No Carb Foods?

In the realm of a no-carb diet, understanding what qualifies as no-carb foods is essential for maintaining dietary goals effectively. No-carb foods are defined primarily by their lack of digestible carbohydrates, which means they have negligible or zero impact on blood sugar levels. This dietary approach focuses on excluding foods that contribute to carbohydrate intake while prioritizing those that align with a zero-carb criterion. Foods that fit this profile typically include proteins, fats, and certain low-carb vegetables, each playing a distinct role in a balanced no-carb diet.

Meats and poultry are prime examples of no-carb foods. Beef, chicken, pork, and turkey, when unprocessed and free from added sugars or carb-containing fillers, contain no carbohydrates. These protein sources provide essential nutrients and are central to a no-carb eating plan. The absence of carbohydrates in these foods makes them ideal for creating satisfying and nutrient-dense meals, without impacting blood sugar levels.

Seafood also fits into the no-carb category. Fish such as salmon, tuna, and trout, along with shellfish like shrimp and crab, are naturally free from carbs. These options not only add variety to your diet but also offer valuable omega-3 fatty acids and other nutrients beneficial to overall health. Ensuring that the seafood is fresh and minimally processed will help maintain its no-carb status.

Eggs are another staple in a no-carb diet. Both whole eggs and egg whites are devoid of carbohydrates and serve as a versatile ingredient in many dishes. They are rich in protein and essential vitamins, making them a cornerstone of a no-carb meal plan. Whether used in cooking or baking, eggs can help provide structure and substance to various recipes without introducing carbs.

Cheeses, particularly hard and aged varieties, are typically low in carbs. Cheddar, Parmesan, and similar cheeses contain minimal to zero carbs, depending on their processing. Soft cheeses like cream cheese and ricotta also fit within the no-carb framework, though it is always wise to check labels for any added ingredients that might introduce carbohydrates. Cheese adds flavor and richness to meals, complementing other no-carb foods.

Oils and fats, including olive oil, coconut oil, butter, and avocado oil, are also devoid of carbohydrates. These ingredients are crucial for cooking and adding flavor to meals. They provide energy and can be used to prepare a variety of no-carb dishes. By incorporating these fats into your diet, you can enjoy flavorful meals while adhering to a no-carb lifestyle.

Low-carb vegetables, though not entirely devoid of carbohydrates, are included in a no-carb diet due to their very minimal carb content. Leafy greens such as spinach and kale, cruciferous vegetables like broccoli and cauliflower, and mushrooms fall into this category. These vegetables provide essential nutrients and fiber without significantly affecting your carbohydrate intake, supporting overall health while maintaining dietary goals.

Importance of Reading Nutrition Labels

Reading nutrition labels is a crucial practice when adhering to a no-carb diet, as it ensures that you remain within the dietary guidelines necessary for achieving your health goals. Nutrition labels provide a wealth of information about the carbohydrate content of packaged foods, which is essential for maintaining strict control over your intake. By carefully examining these labels, you can distinguish between foods that fit into your no-carb lifestyle and those that might undermine your efforts.

When analyzing a nutrition label, start by focusing on the total carbohydrate count. This figure is prominently listed and indicates the amount of carbohydrates present in a single serving of the product. For a no-carb diet, it's important to choose foods with as close to zero carbohydrates as possible. Even small amounts of carbs can add up over time, so vigilance is key to avoiding accidental intake that could disrupt your progress.

In addition to the total carbohydrates, scrutinize the breakdown of the types of carbohydrates listed on the label. Pay attention to dietary fiber and sugars. While dietary fiber is not digested in the same way as other carbohydrates, contributing minimally to blood sugar levels, it's still important to consider in the context of a no-carb diet. Similarly, sugars, whether added or naturally occurring, can contribute to your overall carbohydrate intake and should be avoided.

Ingredients lists on nutrition labels are also vital. Ingredients are listed in descending order of quantity, so if a high-carb ingredient, such as flour or sugar, appears near the top, it's a clear indicator that the product may not be suitable for a no-carb diet. Even seemingly healthy products can contain hidden carbs, so a thorough examination of the ingredients list is necessary to ensure compliance with your dietary goals.

It's also beneficial to be aware of serving sizes as indicated on the label. A product that seems low in carbohydrates per serving might still contain significant carbs if the serving size is larger than what you would normally consume. Always compare the serving size to your actual portion to accurately gauge the carbohydrate content of the food you're eating.

Understanding how to read nutrition labels can also help you identify suitable alternatives. For instance, if you find that a particular brand of a product contains too many carbs, you might be able to find a similar product with a lower carbohydrate count. Many brands offer no-carb or low-carb versions of common foods, so being proficient in label reading can aid in finding the best options available.

Overall, the practice of reading nutrition labels empowers you to make informed decisions and maintain adherence to your no-carb diet. By integrating this practice into your shopping routine, you'll enhance your ability to manage your carbohydrate intake effectively, avoid unintentional deviations, and achieve the health benefits associated with a no-carb lifestyle. Understanding and utilizing nutrition labels is not just a task; it's an essential skill for successfully navigating your dietary choices.

Chapter 2: Foods to Eat

Meats and Poultry

Here is a comprehensive table detailing various meats and poultry suitable for a no-carb diet, including ingredient, instructions, nutritional information, serving size, and cooking time:

Meat/ Poultry	Ingredients	Instructions	Nutritional Information	Serving Size	Cooking Time
Beef Sirloin	Beef sirloin steak	Season with salt and pepper, grill or pan-sear to desired doneness	Calories: 225, Protein: 23g, Carbs: 0g, Fat: 15g	6 oz	6-8 minutes per side

Chicke n Breast	Boneles s, skinless chicken breast	Season, bake at 375°F or grill until cooked through	Calories : 165, Protein: 31g, Carbs: 0g, Fat: 3.6g	4 oz	20-25 minutes (bake)
Pork Chops	Bone-in or boneles s pork chops	Season, pan-sea r or bake at 375°F until done	Calories : 231, Protein: 27g, Carbs: 0g, Fat: 14g	6 oz	6-7 minutes per side (pan-sea r)
Groun d Beef	85% lean ground beef	Brown in a pan, season to taste	Calories : 250, Protein: 26g, Carbs: 0g, Fat: 17g	4 oz	6-8 minutes
Turkey Breast	Boneles s, skinless	Season, bake at 375°F	Calories : 135, Protein:	4 oz	25-30 minutes

	turkey breast	until cooked through	30g, Carbs: 0g, Fat: 1g		
Lamb Chops	Lamb chops	Season, grill or pan-sear to preferred doneness	Calories: 282, Protein: 22g, Carbs: 0g, Fat: 21g	6 oz	4-5 minutes per side
Beef Tenderloin	Beef tenderloin steak	Season, grill or pan-sear to desired doneness	Calories: 210, Protein: 23g, Carbs: 0g, Fat: 13g	6 oz	6-8 minutes per side
Chicken Thighs	Boneless, skinless chicken thighs	Season, bake at 375°F or grill	Calories: 209, Protein: 26g, Carbs:	4 oz	25-30 minutes (bake)

		until done	0g, Fat: 10g		
Pork Ribs	Pork ribs	Season, bake or grill until tender	Calories : 250, Protein: 23g, Carbs: 0g, Fat: 20g	6 oz	2-3 hours (bake)
Duck Breast	Duck breast	Season, pan-sear or grill until crispy	Calories : 300, Protein: 20g, Carbs: 0g, Fat: 24g	4 oz	5-6 minutes per side
Ground Turkey	Lean ground turkey	Brown in a pan, season to taste	Calories : 160, Protein: 22g, Carbs: 0g, Fat: 8g	4 oz	6-8 minutes

Beef Brisket	Beef brisket	Season, slow-cook or bake until tender	Calories : 320, Protein: 24g, Carbs: 0g, Fat: 22g	6 oz	3-4 hours (slow-cook)
Chicken Wings	Chicken wings	Season, bake or fry until crispy	Calories : 203, Protein: 18g, Carbs: 0g, Fat: 14g	4 oz	40-45 minutes (bake)
Veal Chops	Veal chops	Season, grill or pan-sear to desired doneness	Calories : 220, Protein: 25g, Carbs: 0g, Fat: 13g	6 oz	4-5 minutes per side
Bacon	Pork bacon	Cook in a pan or bake	Calories : 42 per slice,	1 slice	2-4 minutes

		until crispy	Protein: 3g, Carbs: 0g, Fat: 3g		per side (pan)

This table provides an overview of various meats and poultry options for a no-carb diet, including details on preparation methods and key nutritional information.

Seafood

Here's a detailed comprehensive table about "Seafood" in relation to the No Carb Food List, including 15 seafood ingredients, instructions, nutritional information, serving size, and cooking time:

Seafood Ingredient	Instructions	Nutritional Information (per 3 oz serving)	Serving Size	Cooking Time
Salmon	Grill, bake, or pan-sear with olive oil and seasoning.	Calories: 180, Protein: 22g, Fat: 10g, Carbs: 0g	3 oz	10-15 minutes
Tuna	Grill, sear, or bake with lemon and herbs.	Calories: 110, Protein: 24g, Fat: 1g, Carbs: 0g	3 oz	5-10 minutes

Shrimp	Sauté, grill, or steam with garlic and butter.	Calories: 85, Protein: 20g, Fat: 1g, Carbs: 0g	3 oz	3-5 minutes
Cod	Bake, grill, or steam with lemon and dill.	Calories: 90, Protein: 20g, Fat: 1g, Carbs: 0g	3 oz	10-12 minutes
Crab	Boil or steam and serve with clarified butter.	Calories: 70, Protein: 15g, Fat: 1g, Carbs: 0g	3 oz	10-12 minutes
Lobster	Boil or steam and serve with drawn butter.	Calories: 80, Protein: 17g, Fat: 1g, Carbs: 0g	3 oz	10-15 minutes

Scallops	Sear with olive oil and garlic in a hot pan.	Calories: 95, Protein: 19g, Fat: 1g, Carbs: 0g	3 oz	3-4 minutes
Mahi-Mahi	Grill, bake, or pan-sear with tropical spices.	Calories: 100, Protein: 22g, Fat: 1g, Carbs: 0g	3 oz	10-12 minutes
Halibut	Bake, grill, or pan-sear with herbs and lemon.	Calories: 110, Protein: 23g, Fat: 2g, Carbs: 0g	3 oz	10-15 minutes
Sardines	Grill or bake with olive oil and herbs.	Calories: 180, Protein: 20g, Fat: 10g, Carbs: 0g	3 oz	5-7 minutes

Clams	Steam with white wine and garlic.	Calories: 75, Protein: 13g, Fat: 1g, Carbs: 0g	3 oz	5-10 minutes
Mussels	Steam with white wine, garlic, and butter.	Calories: 70, Protein: 12g, Fat: 2g, Carbs: 0g	3 oz	5-10 minutes
Oysters	Grill, steam, or eat raw with lemon juice.	Calories: 60, Protein: 6g, Fat: 2g, Carbs: 0g	3 oz	5-10 minutes
Swordfish	Grill or bake with herbs and olive oil.	Calories: 160, Protein: 22g, Fat: 7g, Carbs: 0g	3 oz	10-15 minutes

| Tilapia | Bake, grill, or pan-sear with seasoning. | Calories: 90, Protein: 20g, Fat: 2g, Carbs: 0g | 3 oz | 10-12 minutes |

This table provides a comprehensive overview of various seafood options suitable for a no-carb diet, along with instructions, nutritional information, serving size, and cooking time. Each entry is designed to help you prepare and enjoy these nutritious, low-carb seafood dishes easily.

Eggs

Here's a detailed and comprehensive content about "Eggs" in relation to the No Carb Food List, presented in a table format:

Dish	Ingredients	Instructions	Nutritional Information (Per Serving)	Serving Size	Cooking Time
1. Scrambled Eggs	3 large eggs, 2 tbsp butter, Salt and pepper to taste	Whisk eggs, melt butter in a pan, pour in eggs, stir gently until cooked.	Calories: 250, Protein: 17g, Fat: 20g, Carbs: 0g	1 serving	5 minutes

| 2. **Boiled Eggs** | 4 large eggs, Water | Place eggs in a pot, cover with water, boil for 10 minutes, cool in ice water. | Calories: 70 (per egg), Protein: 6g, Fat: 5g, Carbs: 0g | 1 egg | 10 minutes |
| 3. **Omelette** | 3 large eggs, 1/4 cup cheese, 1/4 cup diced ham, Salt and pepper to taste | Whisk eggs, pour into heated pan, add cheese and ham, fold omelette when | Calories: 300, Protein: 20g, Fat: 24g, Carbs: 0g | 1 serving | 10 minutes |

		eggs are set.			
4. Poache d Eggs	2 large eggs, Water, 1 tbsp vinegar	Boil water with vinegar, create a whirlpo ol, gently add eggs, cook for 3 minutes .	Calories : 70 (per egg), Protein: 6g, Fat: 5g, Carbs: 0g	2 eggs	5 minutes
5. Devile d Eggs	6 large eggs, 1/4 cup mayonn aise, 1 tsp mustar d, Paprika	Boil and halve eggs, mix yolks with mayonn aise and	Calories : 100, Protein: 7g, Fat: 8g, Carbs: 0g	1 egg	15 minutes

	for garnish	mustard, refill whites, sprinkle paprika.			
6. Egg Salad	4 large eggs, 1/4 cup mayonnaise, 1 tbsp Dijon mustard, Salt and pepper to taste	Boil and chop eggs, mix with mayonnaise and mustard, season with salt and pepper.	Calories: 150, Protein: 10g, Fat: 12g, Carbs: 0g	1 serving	10 minutes
7. Egg Muffins	6 large eggs, 1/2 cup diced vegetables, 1/4	Whisk eggs, add vegetables and cheese,	Calories: 120, Protein: 9g, Fat: 9g,	1 muffin	25 minutes

| | cup cheese, Salt and pepper to taste | pour into muffin tin, bake at 350°F for 20 minutes . | Carbs: 1g | | |
| **8. Cloud Eggs** | 4 large eggs, Salt and pepper to taste | Separate whites from yolks, whip whites to stiff peaks, spoon onto baking sheet, create a well, add yolks, | Calories : 70 (per egg), Protein: 6g, Fat: 5g, Carbs: 0g | 1 egg | 10 minutes |

		bake at 450°F for 5 minutes .			
9. Egg Drop Soup	4 cups chicken broth, 2 large eggs, 1 tbsp soy sauce, 1/4 tsp white pepper	Boil broth with soy sauce and pepper, whisk eggs, slowly pour into broth while stirring.	Calories : 50, Protein: 3g, Fat: 3g, Carbs: 1g	1 cup	10 minutes
10. Shaksh uka	4 large eggs, 2 cups tomato sauce,	Sauté onions and peppers , add	Calories : 120, Protein: 6g, Fat: 7g,	1 serving	20 minutes

	1/2 cup bell peppers, 1/4 cup onions, 1 tsp cumin	tomato sauce and cumin, make wells, crack eggs into wells, cook until eggs are set.	Carbs: 5g		
11. Baked Eggs in Avocado	2 large eggs, 1 avocado, Salt and pepper to taste	Halve and pit avocado, crack egg into each half, bake at 425°F for 15	Calories: 200, Protein: 6g, Fat: 18g, Carbs: 2g	1 serving	20 minutes

		minutes.			
12. Egg and Cheese Cups	6 large eggs, 1/2 cup shredded cheese, Salt and pepper to taste	Whisk eggs, mix in cheese, pour into greased muffin tin, bake at 350°F for 15 minutes.	Calories: 120, Protein: 9g, Fat: 9g, Carbs: 0g	1 cup	20 minutes
13. Frittata	6 large eggs, 1/2 cup diced vegetables, 1/4 cup cheese, Salt and	Whisk eggs, add vegetables and cheese, pour into oven-saf	Calories: 200, Protein: 12g, Fat: 15g, Carbs: 2g	1 slice	20 minutes

	pepper to taste	e pan, cook on stove until set, broil for 2 minutes .			
14. Egg Curry	4 large eggs, 1 cup coconut milk, 1/2 cup diced tomatoes, 1 tbsp curry powder	Boil eggs, sauté tomatoes with curry powder, add coconut milk, simmer, add eggs, cook for 10	Calories: 180, Protein: 7g, Fat: 14g, Carbs: 3g	1 serving	20 minutes

		minutes.			
15. Scotch Eggs	4 large eggs, 1/2 lb sausage meat, Salt and pepper to taste	Boil and peel eggs, wrap in sausage meat, bake at 400°F for 20 minutes.	Calories: 250, Protein: 15g, Fat: 20g, Carbs: 1g	1 egg	30 minutes

Eggs are a versatile and nutrient-dense food that fit perfectly into a no-carb diet. By including a variety of egg-based dishes in your meal plans, you can enjoy a range of flavors and textures while adhering to your dietary goals.

Cheeses

Here's a detailed comprehensive content about "Cheeses" for a no-carb food list, including ingredients, instructions, nutritional information, serving size, and cooking time, presented in a table format:

Cheese	Ingredients	Instructions	Nutritional Information (per 1 oz)	Serving Size	Cooking Time
Cheddar	Milk, Salt, Enzymes	Slice or cube for snacks or melt over dishes.	Calories: 110, Fat: 9g, Protein: 7g, Carbs: 0g	1 oz (28g)	5-10 minutes (melting)
Parmesan	Milk, Salt, Enzymes	Grate over salads or pasta	Calories: 110, Fat: 7g, Protein: 10g,	1 oz (28g)	No cooking needed

		alternatives.	Carbs: 0g		
Mozzarella	Milk, Salt, Enzymes	Slice for salads or melt on pizza alternatives.	Calories: 85, Fat: 6g, Protein: 6g, Carbs: 0g	1 oz (28g)	5-10 minutes (melting)
Swiss	Milk, Salt, Enzymes	Slice for sandwiches or melt in recipes.	Calories: 106, Fat: 8g, Protein: 8g, Carbs: 0g	1 oz (28g)	5-10 minutes (melting)
Gouda	Milk, Salt, Enzymes	Slice for snacking or melt in recipes.	Calories: 110, Fat: 9g, Protein: 7g, Carbs: 0g	1 oz (28g)	5-10 minutes (melting)

Blue Cheese	Milk, Salt, Enzymes, Cultures	Crumble over salads or use in dressings.	Calories: 100, Fat: 8g, Protein: 6g, Carbs: 0g	1 oz (28g)	No cooking needed
Feta	Milk, Salt, Enzymes	Crumble over salads or use in Greek dishes.	Calories: 75, Fat: 6g, Protein: 4g, Carbs: 0g	1 oz (28g)	No cooking needed
Brie	Milk, Salt, Enzymes	Slice for cheese boards or bake for appetizers.	Calories: 95, Fat: 8g, Protein: 6g, Carbs: 0g	1 oz (28g)	10-15 minutes (baking)
Goat Cheese	Goat Milk, Salt,	Spread on crackers	Calories: 75, Fat: 6g,	1 oz (28g)	No cooking needed

	Enzymes	or crumble over salads.	Protein: 5g, Carbs: 0g		
Colby Jack	Milk, Salt, Enzymes	Slice for sandwiches or melt in recipes.	Calories: 110, Fat: 9g, Protein: 7g, Carbs: 0g	1 oz (28g)	5-10 minutes (melting)
Provolone	Milk, Salt, Enzymes	Slice for sandwiches or melt in recipes.	Calories: 98, Fat: 7g, Protein: 7g, Carbs: 0g	1 oz (28g)	5-10 minutes (melting)
Havarti	Milk, Salt, Enzymes	Slice for sandwiches or melt in recipes.	Calories: 105, Fat: 8g, Protein: 6g,	1 oz (28g)	5-10 minutes (melting)

			Carbs: 0g		
Ricotta	Milk, Salt, Enzymes	Use in lasagna or desserts.	Calories: 90, Fat: 7g, Protein: 6g, Carbs: 0g	1 oz (28g)	30-40 minutes (baking)
Cream Cheese	Milk, Cream, Salt, Enzymes	Spread on low-carb bread or use in recipes.	Calories: 100, Fat: 9g, Protein: 2g, Carbs: 0g	1 oz (28g)	No cooking needed
Asiago	Milk, Salt, Enzymes	Grate over dishes or slice for snacking.	Calories: 110, Fat: 9g, Protein: 7g, Carbs: 0g	1 oz (28g)	No cooking needed

These cheeses are perfect for a no-carb diet and can be enjoyed in a variety of ways. Whether you're looking to melt cheese over a dish, crumble it over a salad, or simply enjoy it as a snack, each option offers delicious flavor and nutritional benefits without the carbs. Incorporate these cheeses into your meals to enhance flavor while maintaining your dietary goals.

Oils and Fats

Here's a detailed comprehensive content about "Oils and Fats" in relation to the No Carb Food List, formatted as a table:

Ingredient	Instructions	Nutritional Information (per tablespoon)	Serving Size	Cooking Time
Olive Oil	Use for salad dressings, sautéing vegetables, or drizzling over finished dishes.	120 calories, 14g fat, 0g carbs, 0g protein	1 tablespoon	Varies
Coconut Oil	Ideal for frying, baking, or adding to	121 calories, 13.5g fat,	1 tablespoon	Varies

	smoothies and coffee for a rich, creamy texture.	0g carbs, 0g protein		
Avocado Oil	Perfect for high-heat cooking, roasting vegetables, or as a base for homemade mayonnaise.	124 calories, 14g fat, 0g carbs, 0g protein	1 tablespoon	Varies
Butter	Use for sautéing, baking, or melting over vegetables and meats for added flavor.	102 calories, 12g fat, 0g carbs, 0g protein	1 tablespoon	Varies

Ghee	Great for frying, roasting, or adding to coffee for a no-carb, energy-boosting beverage.	112 calories, 13g fat, 0g carbs, 0g protein	1 tablespoon	Varies
Lard	Use for frying, baking, or adding to soups and stews for richness.	115 calories, 13g fat, 0g carbs, 0g protein	1 tablespoon	Varies
Tallow	Ideal for deep frying, roasting, and adding flavor to	115 calories, 13g fat, 0g carbs, 0g protein	1 tablespoon	Varies

	savory dishes.			
Bacon Fat	Use for frying eggs, sautéing greens, or adding a smoky flavor to various dishes.	115 calories, 13g fat, 0g carbs, 0g protein	1 tablespoo n	Varies
Duck Fat	Perfect for roasting potatoes, frying, or making confit.	113 calories, 13g fat, 0g carbs, 0g protein	1 tablespoo n	Varies
Macadami a Oil	Excellent for salad dressings, baking, or low-heat cooking.	120 calories, 14g fat, 0g carbs, 0g protein	1 tablespoo n	Varies

Almond Oil	Best used for low-heat cooking, baking, or adding to salad dressings.	120 calories, 14g fat, 0g carbs, 0g protein	1 tablespoon	Varies
Walnut Oil	Ideal for salad dressings, drizzling over finished dishes, or adding to cold dishes.	120 calories, 14g fat, 0g carbs, 0g protein	1 tablespoon	Varies
Sesame Oil	Use for stir-frying, adding to marinades, or drizzling over Asian	120 calories, 14g fat, 0g carbs, 0g protein	1 tablespoon	Varies

	dishes for flavor.			
Flaxseed Oil	Best used for cold dishes, salad dressings, or adding to smoothies.	120 calories, 14g fat, 0g carbs, 0g protein	1 tablespoon	Varies
MCT Oil	Add to coffee, smoothies, or use as a supplement for quick energy.	130 calories, 14g fat, 0g carbs, 0g protein	1 tablespoon	Varies

These oils and fats are integral to a no-carb diet, providing essential nutrients and enhancing the flavor of your dishes without adding any carbohydrates. Each type of oil or fat can be used in a variety of cooking methods, from frying and baking to dressing and drizzling, making them versatile and valuable staples in your kitchen.

Low Carb Vegetables (Minimal Carbs)

Here's a detailed table on "Low Carb Vegetables (Minimal Carbs)" for the No Carb Food List, including 15 low carb vegetables with their ingredients, instructions, nutritional information, serving sizes, and cooking times.

Vegetable	Ingredients	Instructions	Nutritional Information	Serving Size	Cooking Time
Spinach	Fresh spinach leaves	Rinse and chop leaves. Sauté with olive oil and garlic for 2-3 minutes.	1g carbs, 0.5g fiber, 0.5g net carbs	1 cup (30g)	2-3 minutes (sautéed)

Kale	Fresh kale leaves	Rinse, chop, and massage with olive oil. Bake at 350°F for 10-15 minutes for kale chips.	1.4g carbs, 0.6g fiber, 0.8g net carbs	1 cup (20g)	10-15 minutes (baked)
Broccoli	Broccoli florets	Steam florets for 5-7 minutes until tender.	6g carbs, 2.4g fiber, 3.6g net carbs	1 cup (91g)	5-7 minutes (steamed)
Cauliflower	Cauliflower florets	Steam or roast florets for 20-25	5g carbs, 2g fiber, 3g net carbs	1 cup (107g)	20-25 minutes (roasted)

		minutes until tender.			
Zucchini	Sliced zucchini	Sauté slices with olive oil and herbs for 4-5 minutes.	3.5g carbs, 1g fiber, 2.5g net carbs	1 cup (124g)	4-5 minutes (sautéed)
Bell Peppers	Sliced bell peppers	Sauté or roast slices for 10-12 minutes until tender.	6g carbs, 2g fiber, 4g net carbs	1 cup (92g)	10-12 minutes (roasted)
Mushrooms	Sliced mushrooms	Sauté with garlic and	2.3g carbs, 1g fiber,	1 cup (70g)	5-7 minutes (sautéed)

		olive oil for 5-7 minutes.	1.3g net carbs		
Aspara gus	Fresh asparag us spears	Steam or grill for 5-10 minutes until tender.	5g carbs, 2.8g fiber, 2.2g net carbs	1 cup (134g)	5-10 minutes (grilled)
Avocad o	Halved avocado	Serve raw or add to salads and dishes.	12g carbs, 10g fiber, 2g net carbs	1 cup (150g)	No cooking require d
Cucum ber	Sliced cucum ber	Serve raw in salads or as snacks.	3.8g carbs, 1g fiber, 2.8g net carbs	1 cup (104g)	No cooking require d

Lettuce	Fresh lettuce leaves	Rinse and chop leaves for salads or wraps.	2g carbs, 1g fiber, 1g net carbs	1 cup (36g)	No cooking required
Green Beans	Fresh green beans	Steam or boil for 5-7 minutes until tender.	7g carbs, 3.4g fiber, 3.6g net carbs	1 cup (125g)	5-7 minutes (steamed)
Celery	Chopped celery stalks	Serve raw with dips or in salads.	3g carbs, 1.6g fiber, 1.4g net carbs	1 cup (101g)	No cooking required
Radishes	Sliced radishes	Serve raw in salads or roast	4g carbs, 2g fiber,	1 cup (116g)	15-20 minutes (roasted)

		for 15-20 minutes.	2g net carbs		
Brussels Sprouts	Halved Brussels sprouts	Roast with olive oil and salt for 25-30 minutes until crispy.	8g carbs, 3.3g fiber, 4.7g net carbs	1 cup (88g)	25-30 minutes (roasted)

These low carb vegetables can be incorporated into your no-carb diet plan, providing essential nutrients while keeping your carbohydrate intake minimal. Adjust serving sizes and cooking times based on your preferences and the specific recipes you follow.

Beverages

Here's a detailed table with 15 no-carb beverages, including ingredients, instructions, nutritional information, serving size, and cooking time:

Beverage	Ingredients	Instructions	Nutritional Information (per serving)	Serving Size	Cooking Time
Black Coffee	1 cup water, 1 tbsp coffee grounds	Brew coffee using your preferred method (drip, French press, etc.)	0g carbs, 2 calories, 0g fat, 0g protein	8 fl oz	5 mins

Green Tea	1 cup water, 1 green tea bag	Boil water, steep tea bag for 3-5 minutes	0g carbs, 0 calories, 0g fat, 0g protein	8 fl oz	5 mins
Herbal Tea	1 cup water, 1 herbal tea bag (e.g., peppermint, chamomile)	Boil water, steep tea bag for 5-7 minutes	0g carbs, 0 calories, 0g fat, 0g protein	8 fl oz	5 mins
Sparkling Water	1 cup sparkling water, lemon or lime wedge	Pour sparkling water into a glass, add a wedge of lemon or lime	0g carbs, 0 calories, 0g fat, 0g protein	8 fl oz	1 min

Iced Coffee	1 cup brewed coffee, ice cubes	Brew coffee, let it cool, pour over ice	0g carbs, 2 calories, 0g fat, 0g protein	8 fl oz	10 mins
Cold Brew Coffee	1 cup cold water, 1 tbsp coarsely ground coffee	Combine water and coffee grounds, steep in fridge for 12-24 hours, strain	0g carbs, 2 calories, 0g fat, 0g protein	8 fl oz	12-24 hrs (steeping time)
Bone Broth	1 cup bone broth	Heat broth in a pot until warm	0g carbs, 40 calories, 0g fat,	8 fl oz	5 mins

			10g protein		
Infused Water	1 cup water, slices of cucumber or mint leaves	Add cucumber slices or mint leaves to water, let sit for 1 hour	0g carbs, 0 calories, 0g fat, 0g protein	8 fl oz	1 hr
Kombucha (unsweetened)	1 cup unsweetened kombucha	Pour kombucha into a glass and serve chilled	0g carbs, 30 calories, 0g fat, 0g protein	8 fl oz	1 min
Plain Almond Milk	1 cup unsweetened	Pour almond milk into a	1g carbs, 30 calories,	8 fl oz	1 min

	almond milk	glass and serve chilled	2.5g fat, 1g protein		
Coconut Water (unsweetened)	1 cup unsweetened coconut water	Pour coconut water into a glass and serve chilled	2g carbs, 45 calories, 0g fat, 0g protein	8 fl oz	1 min
Electrolyte Water	1 cup water, 1/8 tsp salt, 1/8 tsp baking soda, lemon juice	Mix ingredients in water, stir until dissolved	0g carbs, 0 calories, 0g fat, 0g protein	8 fl oz	2 mins
Matcha Tea	1 cup water, 1 tsp	Boil water, whisk	0g carbs, 0 calories,	8 fl oz	5 mins

	matcha powder	matcha powder in water until frothy	0g fat, 0g protein		
Protein Shake	1 cup water, 1 scoop no-carb protein powder	Mix protein powder with water, shake well	0g carbs, varies by brand (approx. 100 calories, 0g fat, 25g protein)	8 fl oz	2 mins
Bulletproof Coffee	1 cup brewed coffee, 1 tbsp unsalted butter, 1 tbsp	Brew coffee, blend with butter and coconut	0g carbs, 220 calories, 25g fat, 0g protein	8 fl oz	5 mins

	coconut oil	oil until creamy			

These beverages are carefully selected to fit into a no-carb diet, providing hydration and flavor without the addition of unwanted carbohydrates. Each recipe is quick and easy to prepare, ensuring that you can enjoy these drinks with minimal effort.

Condiments and Spices

Here's a detailed and comprehensive table about condiments and spices suitable for a no-carb diet:

Ingredient	Instructions	Nutritional Information	Serving Size	Cooking Time
Salt	Use sparingly to season meats, vegetables, and sauces.	0g carbs, 0 calories, 0g fat	1/4 tsp	N/A
Black Pepper	Grind fresh over dishes for enhanced flavor.	0g carbs, 0 calories, 0g fat	1/4 tsp	N/A
Paprika	Sprinkle over meats,	0g carbs, 0 calories, 0g fat	1/4 tsp	N/A

	vegetables, or eggs for a mild, sweet flavor.			
Turmeric	Use in curries, soups, or as a seasoning for meats and vegetables.	0g carbs, 0 calories, 0g fat	1/4 tsp	N/A
Cayenne Pepper	Add a pinch to dishes for a spicy kick.	0g carbs, 0 calories, 0g fat	1/8 tsp	N/A
Cumin	Use in marinades, rubs, or sprinkle over	0g carbs, 0 calories, 0g fat	1/4 tsp	N/A

	roasted vegetables.			
Garlic Powder	Use in place of fresh garlic for seasoning meats, vegetables, and sauces.	1g carbs, 4 calories, 0g fat	1/4 tsp	N/A
Onion Powder	Add to soups, stews, and rubs for a savory depth.	1g carbs, 4 calories, 0g fat	1/4 tsp	N/A
Oregano	Use dried oregano in Italian dishes, marinades, and sauces.	0g carbs, 0 calories, 0g fat	1/4 tsp	N/A

Basil	Add dried basil to tomato-ba sed dishes, meats, and sauces.	0g carbs, 0 calories, 0g fat	1/4 tsp	N/A
Dill Weed	Sprinkle over fish, chicken, and vegetables for a fresh flavor.	0g carbs, 0 calories, 0g fat	1/4 tsp	N/A
Rosemar y	Use in marinades , rubs, or sprinkle over roasted meats and vegetables.	0g carbs, 0 calories, 0g fat	1/4 tsp	N/A

Thyme	Add to soups, stews, and roasted dishes for an earthy flavor.	0g carbs, 0 calories, 0g fat	1/4 tsp	N/A
Mustard	Use as a condiment for meats and in dressings.	0g carbs, 3 calories, 0g fat	1 tsp	N/A
Hot Sauce	Add to dishes for extra heat; ensure no sugar-added varieties.	0g carbs, 0 calories, 0g fat	1 tsp	N/A
Soy Sauce	Use in marinades and sauces;	1g carbs, 10 calories, 0g fat	1 tbsp	N/A

	opt for low-sodium versions.			
Vinegar	Use in dressings and marinades; options include apple cider, white, and balsamic (check for sugar)	0g carbs, 0 calories, 0g fat (varies with type)	1 tbsp	N/A
Mayonnaise	Use in dressings and as a spread; ensure no sugar-added varieties.	0g carbs, 90 calories, 10g fat	1 tbsp	N/A

| Olive Oil | Use for cooking, dressings, and marinades. | 0g carbs, 120 calories, 14g fat | 1 tbsp | N/A |
| Butter | Use for cooking and as a spread; choose grass-fed for added benefits. | 0g carbs, 100 calories, 11g fat | 1 tbsp | N/A |

This table provides a quick reference to some of the best condiments and spices suitable for a no-carb diet, detailing how to use them, their nutritional information, appropriate serving sizes, and any relevant cooking times. Incorporating these ingredients can greatly enhance the flavor of your meals while keeping your carbohydrate intake in check.

Chapter 3: Foods to Avoid

Sugary Foods

Here's a detailed and comprehensive table about sugary foods that should be avoided on a no-carb diet, including reasons why they should be avoided:

Sugary Food	Description	Reason to Avoid
Candy	Includes chocolates, gummies, hard candies, and licorice.	High in simple sugars, leading to spikes in blood glucose and insulin levels, contributing to weight gain and cravings.
Pastries	Encompasses items like donuts, croissants, danishes, and muffins.	Made with refined flour and sugars, causing rapid increases in blood sugar and providing little nutritional value.

Cakes and Pies	Sweet desserts often consumed during celebrations.	High sugar and carbohydrate content that can disrupt ketosis and contribute to weight gain and metabolic issues.
Ice Cream	Frozen dessert made from dairy and sugar.	Contains significant amounts of added sugars, leading to increased calorie intake and blood sugar fluctuations.
Sugary Drinks	Includes sodas, sweetened teas, energy drinks, and sports drinks.	High in added sugars and empty calories, causing rapid spikes in blood sugar and increased risk of metabolic syndrome.

Cookies and Biscuits	Baked goods often high in sugar and refined flour.	Loaded with sugars and unhealthy fats, which can interfere with weight loss and cause insulin resistance.
Sweetened Yogurts	Yogurts with added sugars and fruit flavorings.	Although marketed as healthy, these contain hidden sugars that can disrupt no-carb dietary goals and increase carb intake.
Granola Bars	Often perceived as a healthy snack but usually high in sugars and carbohydrates.	Contains added sugars and often high in carbohydrates, which can prevent the body from staying in a no-carb state.

Breakfast Cereals	Includes many commercial cereals marketed to children and adults.	Typically high in sugars and refined grains, leading to energy crashes and increased hunger throughout the day.
Syrups	Such as maple syrup, corn syrup, and flavored syrups.	Extremely high in sugars, which can rapidly increase blood sugar levels and provide excess calories with little nutrition.
Sweetened Condiments	Ketchup, barbecue sauce, sweet salad dressings, and similar products.	These condiments contain hidden sugars that can add unnecessary carbs to meals and disrupt ketosis.
Fruit Juices	Includes 100% fruit juices and juice cocktails.	High in natural sugars and lacking the fiber found in whole fruit,

		leading to quick spikes in blood sugar.
Jams and Jellies	Preserved fruit spreads typically high in added sugars.	Contain large amounts of sugar, which can quickly elevate blood sugar levels and disrupt a no-carb diet.
Chocolate Milk	Milk with added chocolate and sugar.	High in sugars and carbohydrates, which can prevent the maintenance of a no-carb dietary state.
Frozen Desserts	Includes items like popsicles, sorbets, and frozen yogurt.	Often loaded with sugars, leading to quick spikes in blood glucose and contributing to excess calorie intake.

This table serves as a comprehensive guide to understanding which sugary foods to avoid on a no-carb diet and the reasons behind these recommendations. Avoiding these foods helps in maintaining stable blood sugar levels, reducing cravings, and promoting overall health and weight management.

Starches and Grains

Here's a detailed and comprehensive table about starches and grains that should be avoided on a no-carb diet:

Ingredient	Description	Reason to Avoid
Bread	Includes white, whole wheat, rye, and other varieties of bread commonly used for sandwiches and toast.	High in carbohydrates, with even whole grain varieties containing significant amounts of starch that can spike blood sugar levels and hinder ketosis.
Pasta	Made from wheat, rice, or other grains; includes spaghetti, macaroni, noodles, and other forms of pasta.	Extremely high in carbohydrates, making it difficult to maintain a low or no-carb diet and can lead to blood sugar spikes.

Rice	Includes white rice, brown rice, wild rice, and other varieties.	High carbohydrate content, even in whole grain varieties like brown rice, which can disrupt ketosis and elevate blood sugar levels.
Cereal	Breakfast cereals, including those marketed as healthy options like granola and oatmeal.	Typically high in sugar and starch, even those labeled as healthy or whole grain, which can cause significant carbohydrate intake.
Potatoes	Includes white potatoes, sweet potatoes, yams, and other starchy tubers.	High in starch and carbohydrates, leading to rapid increases in blood sugar and insulin levels, counteracting the goals of a no-carb diet.

Corn	Includes whole corn, cornmeal, corn tortillas, and other corn-based products.	High in carbohydrates and often used as a base for other high-carb processed foods, making it difficult to stay within no-carb guidelines.
Quinoa	A grain-like seed often used as a rice substitute.	Although it is a high-protein grain, it still contains a significant amount of carbohydrates, which can interfere with maintaining ketosis.
Barley	A whole grain often used in soups, stews, and as a base for salads.	High carbohydrate content, which can disrupt blood sugar levels and hinder the maintenance of a no-carb diet.

Oats	Includes rolled oats, steel-cut oats, and instant oatmeal.	Despite being a whole grain, oats contain substantial carbohydrates, making them unsuitable for a no-carb diet.
Tortillas	Includes flour and corn tortillas commonly used for wraps and tacos.	High in carbohydrates, with even whole grain varieties contributing significant amounts of starch to the diet.
Bagels	Dense bread products often consumed for breakfast.	Very high in carbohydrates and starch, which can lead to quick spikes in blood sugar levels and contribute to excessive carbohydrate intake.

Crackers	Includes whole grain, wheat, and flavored varieties often used as snacks.	High in carbohydrates, even in small serving sizes, which can easily add up and disrupt a no-carb diet plan.
Pretzels	Baked snack items made from wheat flour.	High carbohydrate content and often consumed in large quantities, leading to significant intake of starches and sugars.
Muffins	Includes bran, corn, and fruit muffins typically consumed for breakfast or snacks.	High in carbohydrates and sugars, which can lead to blood sugar spikes and contribute to high carbohydrate intake.
Couscous	A grain product often used as a side	High in carbohydrates and

	dish or in salads, made from crushed durum wheat.	starch, making it incompatible with a no-carb diet and can interfere with maintaining stable blood sugar levels.
Millet	A small-seeded grain often used in baking and as a cereal alternative.	Despite being a whole grain, it is high in carbohydrates, which can disrupt ketosis and elevate blood sugar levels.

This table provides a clear overview of various starches and grains to avoid when following a no-carb diet. Each item is explained in terms of its composition and the reasons it should be excluded to help maintain the dietary restrictions and achieve the desired health outcomes associated with a no-carb lifestyle.

Fruits

Here's a detailed and comprehensive table about fruits that should be avoided on a no-carb diet and the reasons why:

Fruit	Reason to Avoid
Bananas	High in carbohydrates and natural sugars, bananas can quickly increase your daily carb intake, hindering the goals of a no-carb diet. A medium banana contains approximately 27 grams of carbs.
Apples	Apples are rich in natural sugars and carbs, with one medium apple containing about 25 grams of carbohydrates. Consuming apples can lead to an unintended increase in carb intake.
Oranges	Although oranges are a good source of vitamin C, they

	contain around 15 grams of carbs per medium-sized fruit, making them unsuitable for a no-carb diet.
Grapes	Grapes are particularly high in sugars and carbs, with one cup of grapes containing about 27 grams of carbohydrates. Their small size and sweet taste can make it easy to overconsume them.
Mangoes	Mangoes are among the highest-carb fruits, with one cup of sliced mango containing approximately 25 grams of carbs. Their high sugar content can interfere with maintaining a no-carb diet.
Pineapple	Pineapples are sweet and tropical but contain about 21 grams of carbs per cup. Their high sugar content can quickly add up, making them

	unsuitable for a no-carb regimen.
Cherries	Cherries are packed with natural sugars and carbohydrates, with one cup containing around 22 grams of carbs. They are also easy to overeat due to their small size and appealing taste.
Pears	One medium pear contains about 27 grams of carbs, making them too high in sugars for a no-carb diet. Their natural sweetness contributes significantly to carb intake.
Peaches	Although peaches are delicious and nutritious, one medium peach contains approximately 15 grams of carbs, which can add up quickly.

Plums	Plums have about 8 grams of carbs per small fruit, and their small size can lead to overconsumption, increasing your daily carb intake unintentionally.
Watermelon	Despite being refreshing, watermelon contains about 11 grams of carbs per cup. Its high water content can make it seem harmless, but the carbs add up.
Berries (Mixed)	While some berries are lower in carbs than other fruits, they still contain enough carbs to be restricted on a no-carb diet. For example, one cup of strawberries contains around 12 grams of carbs.
Kiwifruit	Kiwifruit contains about 10 grams of carbs per fruit. Its sweet and tangy flavor masks its relatively high carb content.

Figs	Fresh figs are particularly high in carbs, with one medium fig containing approximately 10 grams of carbohydrates. Their dense texture and sweetness can significantly impact your carb intake.
Papaya	Papaya contains about 15 grams of carbs per cup of cubed fruit. Its sweet flavor and soft texture can make it easy to consume more than intended.

This table highlights the fruits that should be avoided on a no-carb diet and provides the reasons why these fruits are not suitable due to their high carbohydrate and sugar content. By steering clear of these fruits, you can better maintain the guidelines of a no-carb diet and work towards your health and fitness goals effectively.

High Carb Vegetables

Here's a detailed and comprehensive table about high-carb vegetables and why they should be avoided in a no-carb diet:

Vegetable	Carbohydrate Content	Reasons to Avoid
Potatoes	37g carbs per 1 medium potato (173g)	Potatoes are very high in starch and carbohydrates, which can spike blood sugar levels and hinder ketosis. They lack fiber to balance out the high carb content.
Sweet Potatoes	27g carbs per 1 medium sweet potato (130g)	Although they contain more vitamins than regular potatoes, sweet potatoes still have a high carbohydrate content that can

		disrupt a no-carb diet and lead to blood sugar spikes.
Corn	27g carbs per 1 cup (145g)	Corn is a starchy vegetable with a high glycemic index, leading to rapid increases in blood sugar levels. It is also relatively low in fiber.
Peas	21g carbs per 1 cup (160g)	Peas contain both starch and natural sugars, making them unsuitable for a no-carb diet due to their potential to raise blood sugar levels.
Beets	13g carbs per 1 cup (136g)	Beets have a high sugar content, which can lead to increased blood sugar levels. They

		are also rich in natural sugars, making them less ideal for a no-carb diet.
Carrots	12g carbs per 1 cup (128g)	Carrots contain more natural sugars compared to other vegetables, which can contribute to higher carbohydrate intake and affect blood sugar stability.
Butternut Squash	16g carbs per 1 cup (140g)	This winter squash is rich in starch and sugars, leading to a high carbohydrate content that can disrupt a no-carb dietary regimen.

Parsnips	24g carbs per 1 cup (133g)	Parsnips are root vegetables high in starch and natural sugars, which can elevate blood sugar levels and interfere with ketosis.
Pumpkin	12g carbs per 1 cup (245g)	Despite its fiber content, pumpkin is high in natural sugars and carbs, making it less suitable for those on a strict no-carb diet.
Acorn Squash	15g carbs per 1 cup (205g)	Acorn squash contains significant amounts of starch, leading to high carbohydrate content that can prevent the maintenance of ketosis.

Yams	42g carbs per 1 cup (136g)	Yams are similar to sweet potatoes with a high starch content, contributing to increased blood sugar levels and disrupting a no-carb diet.
Plantains	48g carbs per 1 cup (154g)	Plantains are very high in starch and natural sugars, making them unsuitable for a no-carb diet as they can quickly elevate blood sugar levels.
Green Peas	21g carbs per 1 cup (160g)	Green peas contain both starch and sugars, which can lead to high carbohydrate intake and interfere with the

		goals of a no-carb diet.
Lentils	40g carbs per 1 cup (198g)	While rich in protein and fiber, lentils are also high in carbohydrates, making them incompatible with a no-carb diet plan.
Chickpeas	45g carbs per 1 cup (164g)	Chickpeas are legumes with high carbohydrate content, particularly starch, which can significantly increase carb intake and affect blood sugar levels.

This table highlights high-carb vegetables and explains why they should be avoided in a no-carb diet. Each entry details the carbohydrate content and the reasons why these vegetables can hinder your dietary goals, emphasizing the importance of choosing low-carb alternatives to maintain a strict no-carb regimen.

Legumes

Here's a detailed and comprehensive table about legumes and why they should be avoided in a no-carb diet:

Legume	Why to Avoid	Carbohydrate Content	Other Nutritional Information
Black Beans	High in carbohydrates, which can spike blood sugar levels and disrupt ketosis.	40g per cup (cooked)	227 calories, 15g protein, 0.9g fat, 15g fiber
Lentils	High in carbs, making it difficult to maintain a state of ketosis.	40g per cup (cooked)	230 calories, 18g protein, 0.8g fat, 16g fiber
Chickpeas	Significant carbohydrate	45g per cup (cooked)	269 calories, 14.5g

	content can interfere with blood sugar management.		protein, 4.2g fat, 12.5g fiber
Kidney Beans	High in carbs, leading to increased blood sugar and insulin response.	40g per cup (cooked)	225 calories, 15g protein, 0.9g fat, 11g fiber
Pinto Beans	Their high carbohydrate content is unsuitable for a no-carb diet.	45g per cup (cooked)	245 calories, 15g protein, 1.2g fat, 15g fiber
Navy Beans	High carbs content can prevent entering or maintaining ketosis.	47g per cup (cooked)	255 calories, 15g protein, 1.1g fat, 19g fiber

Lima Beans	Carbohydrate-rich, causing spikes in blood glucose levels.	39g per cup (cooked)	209 calories, 11g protein, 0.7g fat, 13g fiber
Peas	Despite being vegetables, peas are high in carbs and should be avoided.	21g per cup (cooked)	134 calories, 8.6g protein, 0.4g fat, 8.8g fiber
Black-eyed Peas	High carbohydrate content can hinder weight loss and blood sugar stability.	35g per cup (cooked)	198 calories, 13g protein, 0.9g fat, 11g fiber
Mung Beans	Elevated carb levels make them unsuitable	39g per cup (cooked)	212 calories, 14g protein, 0.8g fat, 15g fiber

	for a no-carb diet.		
Soybeans	Even though lower in carbs than other legumes, their carb content can still disrupt ketosis.	14g per cup (cooked)	298 calories, 28.6g protein, 15.4g fat, 10.3g fiber
Adzuki Beans	Their high carbohydrate content can prevent entering ketosis.	57g per cup (cooked)	294 calories, 17.3g protein, 0.2g fat, 16.8g fiber
Fava Beans	Significant carb content makes them unsuitable for a no-carb diet.	33g per cup (cooked)	187 calories, 12.9g protein, 0.7g fat, 9.2g fiber

Green Beans	Although lower in carbs, larger quantities can add up and disrupt carb balance.	10g per cup (cooked)	44 calories, 2.4g protein, 0.3g fat, 4g fiber
Broad Beans	High in carbs, making it difficult to stay within no-carb dietary limits.	33g per cup (cooked)	187 calories, 13g protein, 0.7g fat, 9g fiber

This table highlights the legumes that should be avoided on a no-carb diet due to their high carbohydrate content. Including these foods in your diet can disrupt blood sugar levels and prevent you from maintaining ketosis, which is essential for a no-carb lifestyle.

Dairy Products with High Carbs

Here's a detailed and comprehensive table about dairy products with high carbs and why they should be avoided on a no-carb diet:

Dairy Product	Carb Content per Serving	Reason to Avoid
Milk (whole, 2%, skim)	12g carbs per cup	Milk contains lactose, a natural sugar, which contributes significantly to its carb content. This can disrupt ketosis and increase blood sugar levels.
Flavored Yogurt	15-30g carbs per 6 oz	Flavored yogurts often contain added sugars and fruit purees, which elevate the carb content significantly

		compared to plain, unsweetened yogurt.
Sweetened Condensed Milk	166g carbs per cup	Sweetened condensed milk is highly concentrated with added sugars, making it extremely high in carbohydrates and unsuitable for a no-carb diet.
Ice Cream	20-30g carbs per 1/2 cup	Ice cream is typically made with sugar and other high-carb ingredients. Even "light" versions can still contain significant amounts of sugar and carbs.

Cream Cheese with Additives	Varies, typically 5-10g carbs per 2 tbsp	Some flavored or low-fat cream cheeses contain added sugars and thickeners that increase the carb content, making them less suitable for a no-carb diet.
Cottage Cheese	6g carbs per 1/2 cup	Cottage cheese contains lactose and can also have added starches or sugars, contributing to its carb content. Low-carb diets typically avoid these hidden carbs.
Fruit-Flavored Kefir	20g carbs per 1 cup	Fruit-flavored kefir often includes added sugars and fruit purees, which significantly raise its carbohydrate

		levels compared to plain kefir.
Processed Cheese Products	Varies, typically 2-10g carbs per slice	Processed cheese products, like American cheese slices, often contain added starches and sugars for texture and flavor, increasing their carb content.
Chocolate Milk	24-30g carbs per cup	Chocolate milk includes added sugar for flavor, leading to a high carb content unsuitable for a no-carb diet.
Yogurt Drinks	15-40g carbs per bottle	Many yogurt drinks are sweetened and flavored, contributing to high carbohydrate

		levels. They are not suitable for a no-carb diet due to their sugar content.
Buttermilk	12g carbs per cup	Buttermilk contains lactose and sometimes added sugars, making it higher in carbs compared to other fermented dairy products.
Lactose-Free Milk	12g carbs per cup	Lactose-free milk still contains the same amount of carbs as regular milk because the lactose is broken down into simpler sugars rather than removed.
Frozen Yogurt	20-30g carbs per 1/2 cup	Frozen yogurt typically contains

		added sugars and other high-carb ingredients, similar to ice cream, making it unsuitable for a no-carb diet.
Whipped Topping (Canned or Tub)	3-6g carbs per 2 tbsp	Whipped toppings often contain added sugars and high-fructose corn syrup, increasing their carb content and making them less ideal for a no-carb diet.
Reduced-Fat Dairy Products	Varies, generally higher in carbs due to added fillers	Reduced-fat versions of dairy products often have added sugars and starches to compensate for the texture and flavor lost with fat

		removal, increasing their carb content.

This table outlines various high-carb dairy products and explains why they should be avoided on a no-carb diet. By steering clear of these items, you can better maintain a low carbohydrate intake and achieve the health benefits associated with a no-carb lifestyle.

Processed Foods

Here's a detailed and comprehensive table about processed foods and why they should be avoided on a no-carb diet:

Processed Food	Reasons to Avoid
Bread	High in carbohydrates and often contains added sugars and preservatives.
Pasta	Made from refined grains which are high in carbs and low in nutrients.
Breakfast Cereals	Typically high in sugars and refined carbs, leading to spikes in blood sugar levels.
Snack Bars	Often contain hidden sugars and refined carbohydrates, even those marketed as "healthy".
Chips and Crackers	High in refined carbs, unhealthy fats, and often

	contain artificial additives and preservatives.
Processed Meats	Many contain added sugars, fillers, and preservatives that can add hidden carbs.
Candy and Sweets	Extremely high in sugars and empty calories, causing rapid spikes and crashes in blood sugar.
Instant Noodles	High in refined carbs, unhealthy fats, and often loaded with sodium and preservatives.
Frozen Meals	Often contain added sugars, preservatives, and are high in refined carbohydrates.
Sugary Drinks	Loaded with sugars and empty calories, contributing significantly to daily carb intake.
Flavored Yogurts	Typically contain added sugars and sweeteners,

	increasing carb content significantly.
Fast Food	High in refined carbs, unhealthy fats, sugars, and often contain numerous additives and preservatives.
Granola Bars	Despite a healthy image, many are high in sugars, syrups, and refined carbs.
Processed Cheese	Contains additives, fillers, and sometimes hidden sugars, increasing carb content.
Sauces and Dressings	Many are loaded with sugars, high-fructose corn syrup, and other carbs, even if they don't taste sweet.

This table provides a clear and concise reference for processed foods that should be avoided on a no-carb diet, along with the reasons why they can be detrimental to maintaining a no-carb lifestyle.

Chapter 5: Sample Meal Plans

Breakfast

Bacon and Eggs

- **Ingredients**: 2 slices of bacon, 2 large eggs, salt, and pepper to taste
- **Instructions**: Cook the bacon in a skillet over medium heat until crispy, about 5-7 minutes. Remove bacon and set aside. In the same skillet, cook the eggs to your preference (scrambled, fried, or poached), seasoning with salt and pepper.
- **Nutritional Information**: 0g carbs, 300 calories, 25g fat, 18g protein
- **Serving Size**: 1 serving
- **Cooking Time**: 10 minutes

Lunch

Grilled Chicken Salad

- **Ingredients**: 1 chicken breast, 2 cups mixed greens, 1/4 cup sliced cucumbers, 1/4 cup cherry tomatoes, 1/4 avocado, 2 tbsp olive oil, 1 tbsp apple cider vinegar, salt, and pepper

- **Instructions**: Season chicken breast with salt and pepper, then grill over medium-high heat for 6-7 minutes per side, or until fully cooked. Let rest for 5 minutes, then slice. Toss mixed greens, cucumbers, cherry tomatoes, and avocado with olive oil and vinegar. Top with sliced chicken.
- **Nutritional Information**: 2g carbs, 400 calories, 30g fat, 28g protein
- **Serving Size:** 1 serving
- **Cooking Time**: 15 minutes

Dinner

Garlic Butter Shrimp

- **Ingredients**: 1 lb shrimp, peeled and deveined, 3 cloves garlic, minced, 1/4 cup butter, 1 tbsp lemon juice, salt, pepper, 2 tbsp chopped parsley
- **Instructions**: Melt butter in a large skillet over medium heat. Add garlic and cook until fragrant, about 1 minute. Add shrimp, season with salt and pepper, and cook until pink and opaque, about 3-4 minutes. Stir in lemon juice and parsley before serving.
- **Nutritional Information**: 1g carbs, 320 calories, 24g fat, 25g protein
- **Serving Size**: 2 servings
- **Cooking Time**: 10 minutes

Snacks

Deviled Eggs

- **Ingredients**: 4 large eggs, 2 tbsp mayonnaise, 1 tsp Dijon mustard, salt, pepper, paprika for garnish
- **Instructions**: Hard boil the eggs by placing them in a pot of cold water and bringing it to a boil. Once boiling, turn off the heat and let sit for 12 minutes. Cool eggs in ice water, peel, and halve. Remove yolks, mash with mayonnaise, mustard, salt, and pepper. Spoon mixture back into egg whites and sprinkle with paprika.
- **Nutritional Information**: 1g carbs, 200 calories, 18g fat, 9g protein
- **Serving Size**: 2 servings (4 egg halves per serving)
- **Cooking Time**: 20 minutes

Cheese and Olive Plate

- **Ingredients**: 1/2 cup mixed olives, 2 oz cheddar cheese, sliced
- **Instructions**: Arrange olives and cheese slices on a plate.
- **Nutritional Information**: 1g carbs, 300 calories, 25g fat, 14g protein
- **Serving Size**: 1 serving
- **Cooking Time**: 5 minutes

Conclusion

Adopting a no-carb diet requires commitment and a clear understanding of what foods to eat and avoid. By following the guidance in the No Carb Food List, you can navigate this dietary change with confidence. The food lists and detailed explanations provided help ensure that you make informed choices, minimizing the risk of inadvertently consuming hidden carbohydrates. This structured approach allows you to fully embrace the benefits of a no-carb lifestyle.

The No Carb Food List offers a wealth of practical advice and comprehensive information, making the transition to a no-carb diet more manageable. With clear categories of foods to include and exclude, meal planning becomes straightforward and less overwhelming. This clarity is crucial for maintaining consistency and achieving the desired health outcomes, such as weight loss, improved energy levels, and better metabolic health.

Understanding the importance of reading nutrition labels is a key aspect of the no-carb journey. By developing the habit of scrutinizing food labels, you can avoid hidden carbs and make smarter dietary choices. This skill empowers you to maintain strict adherence to your no-carb goals, ensuring that your efforts are not undermined by unintentional consumption of carbohydrates.

Incorporating condiments and spices into your meals adds flavor and variety without compromising your no-carb principles. The No Carb Food List includes a diverse range of these ingredients, allowing you to enjoy delicious, satisfying meals. This variety is essential for preventing dietary boredom and maintaining long-term commitment to the no-carb lifestyle.

Avoiding processed foods is another critical component of a successful no-carb diet. These foods often contain hidden sugars, refined carbs, and unhealthy additives that can derail your progress. By focusing on whole, unprocessed foods as outlined in the No Carb Food List, you can avoid these pitfalls and support your overall health and well-being.

Sample meal plans provided in the No Carb Food List offer practical guidance and inspiration for daily meals. These plans showcase how to create balanced, nutritious, and enjoyable meals that align with your no-carb goals. By following these examples, you can simplify meal preparation and ensure that your diet remains varied and interesting.

The journey to a no-carb lifestyle is a personal and transformative experience. With the comprehensive information and practical tools provided by the No Carb Food List, you are well-equipped to make this journey successful. Embrace the guidance offered, stay committed to your goals, and enjoy the myriad benefits that come with a no-carb way of eating.

9 798334 339200